21- Day Daniel Fast Recipes
Praying Your Way Through to Live Healthy

Author

Vickie H. Benson. Ed.

ISBN-13:978-1542368742

ISBN-10:154236874X

A Healthier You w/Dr. V. Benson
21- Day Daniel Fast Recipes

Table Content

Introduction

We go to God with many requests. We ask Him for forgiveness through secret prayer, confessing our sins, and commit to doing the right thing for the rest our lives. But we fall short of those promises and must start over again with the same prayer because we want let old habits die. That is why He sent His Son, Jesus Christ, to save us from our sins. God knows our flesh is weak. He has already forgiven our sins before we commit them. Thank you, God, for forgiving us for sins known and unknown. So, as we move through this 21-day of fasting and praying, let's ask God to help us with every area of our lives.

Prayer of supplication and fasting is how we are reminded of God's faithfulness and promises with daily scriptures. There are many prayers throughout the Bible to help us during this time of fasting. A prayer of supplication is simply petitioning God or making a request to God on our behalf and on the behalf of others. It is a great idea to pray for others while on the fast through intercession or corporate prayer. Don't be afraid to talk to God. He is our heavenly father. He knows His children. Engage your mind with prayer and meditation, invite God in where ever you are, be faithful to Him, commit to every calling, and know that His word would not return to Him void.

I pray that you allow Jesus Christ to dwell in your life. He is the answer to many of our problems and situations. When the Holy Spirit is present, remain in prayer. You will see God working in your favor.

All we need is faith as the size of a mustard seed and know that He wants what's best for us. Our faith as believers has brought about many changes and blessings when our family commits to 21-days of fasting. The fast is a time of prayer, consecration, and clear focus on God's direction, wisdom, and intervention for our lives.

I have been blessed to introduce this book to you as one of *"A Healthier You"* plans. It is so amazing how the Lord uses His people to direct and help others learn how to incorporate good eating habits. So, while in prayer of supplication, ask God to give you the ability to learn how to eat healthy foods as you cleanse His temple through fasting.

1 Corinthians 6:19 says, *"Don't you realize that your body is the temple of the Holy Spirit, who lives in you and was given to you by God? You do not belong to yourself"*. Pray for God's temple to be cleansed with the renewing of your mind. We are a part of God's body. He wants us to live strong, happy, and healthy.

There is no set day to start the *21-Day Daniel Fast* or a cleanse. Some people start the *21- Day Daniel Fast* on the first day of the year because some are looking to God to make miraculous changes in their life for the new year. These changes may include healing, being more prayerful, a new job, job promotion, building a business, reconciling with family and friends, forgiving others, as well as seeking a connection and closer relationship with God.

In this book, there are 21 days of daily scriptures, 21 delicious planned meals, 21 healthy smoothies, desserts, and snacks to get you through the *21- Day Daniel Fast.* I have added bonus recipes for you and your family to enjoy and a S.M.A.R.T. Goals Chart to carry out your purpose God has for you. *The 21-Daniel Fast* is a time to share with family members Biblical scriptures, prayers, thoughts, and your spiritual walk with God. You also can share your goals in support of your future ambitions. Invite family members and friends on the fast who may not have had the opportunity to try the Daniel Fast before. Prepare the recipes together with family, friends and enjoy the fellowship.

To learn more about eating healthy, detoxing and cleanse please see my website "A Healthier You!" Six Tier Plans. https://www.ahealthieryoudetoxify-cleansewithdrvbenson.org/

Pray this prayer:

Dear Heavenly Father,

Direct my footsteps according to Your plans Lord. I seek you with thanksgiving knowing you will provide all my needs. I pray for others who are in need and let me be a need for others. I believe in your promises and I stand on your promises. Place passion and compassion in my heart to love others. I trust your will be done during this fast as I pray for *(**Fill In**)*. Please don't let me be tempted with sin. I know that I am not perfect, but in my time of imperfection, forgive me. Redeem me Lord, make me a new creature, renew my mind, and renew my strength. Let me walk and talk like you every day. Let everyone I meet see you in me. Lord, as I seek your face; I am certain You will speak to my heart. Help me to live for You. Let the Holy Spirit be present always in all my situations. I surrender and worship you Lord. Be with me, for I know You are omnipresent. Thank You for everlasting and unfailing love for me.

In Jesus name, I pray, Amen.

CHAPTER 1

The Daniel Fast

"I ate no pleasant food, no meat or wine come from my mouth, nor did I anoint myself at all, till three whole weeks were fulfilled" (Daniel 10:2-3 NIV).

Is this your first time fasting? Fasting is a way to abstain from something that is habit forming. The purpose of the *21- Day Daniel Fast* is to give your heart to the Lord while in continuous prayer, building a closer relationship with Him, full-filling a commitment to His will, and abstaining from certain foods.   However, the Daniel Fast is not about the food, but it is about surrendering to God to receive guidance as you seek the Lord with your heart. Hear Him speak to you closely and to stay focus on the true meaning of wanting God to work in your life.

My families first Daniel Fast was not easy. It seemed like every 10 minutes I wanted to eat something to fill my cravings for food I didn't need. I was hungry! I was tempted to eat foods that were not included on the fast. But I kept the faith and remembered how Jesus was tempted while fasting for 40 days and 40 nights. Our flesh is weaker than Jesus and we satisfy our flesh by eating what we want. You will also be tempted. Don't let the flesh take over. Stay in prayer and remain focus.

For many years I have heard about the Daniel Fast, but didn't know the significance of committing to 21-days to loosen the bonds of weakness, the purpose to abstain from certain foods that would bring you closer to God, build stronger faith, and a spiritual walk/relationship with God. I didn't know how to prepare for meals that were allowed on the fast, but I what was destined to eat the right foods, if any, to make the fast meaningful. When I learned the purpose of the Daniel Fast through prayer of supplication, my passion to know God on a deeper level was what I desired.

Once I understood the purpose of the Daniel fast, I started craving the presence of the Lord and stop craving foods I wanted to eat. I started creating my own recipes that kept me in line of God's word. It took some time, but I eventually developed a habit of creating recipes that taste good and healthy. This was the key to a spiritual breakthrough of spiritual healing, and spiritual guidance. After the first day, I realized that God wanted not only to have my heart and mind on Him during the fast, He wanted to show me the abundance of love, peace, prosperity, and keys to maintaining a healthy lifestyle.

Not only have I maintained a healthy lifestyle through detoxing and cleansing, I am committed to stay this way. I am a servant of God; I truly believe He has given us the freedom to make wise choices to keep our body healthy, even with fasting and praying during this period of the Daniel Fast.

I have been doing the Daniel Fast along with my family for 6 years. Between my family and I, we have created numerous of meals, snacks, and desserts to complete the Daniel Fast. However, we have completed the 21 days and sometimes 22 days, if we didn't start on January 1. Sometimes we delayed the Daniel Fast for one or two days to celebrate family member birthdays in January. God knows the heart and He still wants you to turn your plate down, fast and pray while seeking His face for all your needs. I can recall in 2015 our church committed to 40 days of the Daniel Fast. It was a challenge. Well, to make a long story short, we completed the 40 days too. "We can do all things through Christ who strengthens us" *(Philippians 4:13, NIV).*

Prayer is the substance to allow God to intervene in your life to keep you moving through the *21-Day Daniel Fast*. It's not about the food, but to help you increase your spiritual awareness. Rest a sure, when you learn the true meaning of God's purpose for your life, it changes your perspective to live for Him.

CHAPTER 2

21 - Day Daily Scriptures
Prayers and Thoughts

What is your prayer life like? What are your daily thoughts? Did you know if you write your daily thoughts down and search the Bible for the scripture(s), you can easily pray over your situation and prayers will be answered? God has made us promises, and it is okay to remind Him of His promises. I have prayed over my circumstances many times and the results are phenomenal. Even when my prayer life was not as strong as it is now, my connection with God is more vertical than horizontal. I am happy that God has placed me in a position where I can stay focus on purpose and passion that He has given to me. It may have taken some time to come to this realization, but I trust Him with my whole life and I want to stay in His will to reap the benefits of His promises.

Ask God to make your prayer life stronger as you go through the Daniel Fast. Connect with God on a deeper level by writing your thoughts and praying over them. Know that you are having a conversation with Him and He is listening. I have provided 21- Days of Daily Scriptures for meditation. As you meditate on the scriptures daily, repeat them throughout the day. Stay focus, stay positive, and know your purpose and passion. *(If you need more space to write, I have added more space for you at the end of the book).* Use your pen or pencil to write your daily thoughts and speak life into your thoughts. Ask God to increase your knowledge and wisdom.

Day 1 *Daily Scripture and Prayer*

Thessalonians 5:18 - Pray for God's will to be done in our lives, our families and for our Church family.

My Daily Thoughts:

_____

_____

_____

Day 2 *Daily Scripture and Prayer*

Jeremiah 29:11 Pray for God's purposes to be accomplished in our lives.

My Daily Thoughts:

_____

_____

_____

Day 3 *Daily Scripture and Prayer*

Acts 5:12 - Pray for the salvation of your family, friends and colleagues.

My Daily Thoughts:

_____

_____

_____

Day 4 *Daily Scripture and Prayer*

Romans 12: 1-2 - Pray for God's renewal of our minds so we can be a loving church, that we may love each other, and love those that are new to our church.

My Daily Thoughts:

_____

_____

_____

Day 5 *Daily Scripture and Prayer*

2 Corinthians 7:1- Pray for God's forgiveness and purity to be released in our lives for our spiritual growth.

My Daily Thoughts:

_____

_____

_____

Day 6 *Daily Scripture and Prayer*

Luke 4:40 - Pray for healing for all those that are suffering physically, emotionally and psychologically challenged (make a list of people you know that needs prayer. Pray daily for them).

My Daily Thoughts:

_____

_____

_____

Day 7 *Daily Scripture and Prayer*

Philippians 4:19 - Pray for God's provision for those that have unemployed and are facing financial difficulties.

My Daily Thoughts:

_____

_____

_____

Day 8 *Daily Scripture and Prayer*

Ephesians 2:10 - Pray for a heart for missions, to reaches out to the lost. Help us Lord to do what you have called us to do.

My Daily Thoughts:

_____

_____

_____

Day 9 *Daily Scripture and Prayer*

Proverbs 21:1 - Pray for God's wisdom for our government leaders that they may lead in righteousness.

My Daily Thoughts:

_____

_____

_____

Day 10 *Daily Scripture and Prayer*

John 16:8-9 - Pray for God's Salvation to come to those who have yet to take the step of faith.

My Daily Thoughts:

_____

_____

Day 11 *Daily Scripture and Prayer*

Chronicles 7:14 - Pray that God will heal our land, our city, and our economy as we seek Him in prayer.

My Daily Thoughts:

_____

_____

_____

Day 12 *Daily Scripture and Prayer*

Ephesians 4:11- 13 - Pray for our Pastor's and ministry leaders, and worship leaders, that they receive wisdom and knowledge as they lead our churches.

My Daily Thoughts:

_____

_____

Day 13 *Daily Scripture and Prayer*

Romans 10: 14-15 - Pray for our marriages and family ministries. Pray for our church families Pray for families living in all states and nation.

My Daily Thoughts:

_____

_____

Day 14 *Daily Scripture and Prayer*

Exodus 15:26 - Pray that God's word would bring salvation, deliverance, healing, reverse of chronic illnesses and diseases.

My Daily Thoughts:

_____

_____

Day 15 *Daily Scripture and Prayer*

John 16:33 - Pray for God's Love & Peace to cover our relationships, that we may live in harmony with each other.

My Daily Thoughts:

_____

_____

_____

Day 16 *Daily Scripture and Prayer*

1 John, 4:1- Pray that we would share God's love with our families, neighbors, school's colleges/universities, and businesses.

My Daily Thoughts:

_____

_____

Day 17 *Daily Scripture and Prayer*

1 Peter 4:10 - Pray for our ministry volunteers. Pray for strength, resources, provisions as they are doing God's will by serving others.

My Daily Thoughts:

Day 18 *Daily Scripture and Prayer*

Deuteronomy 10:17 -18 - Pray for God's protection for those in our church who are widows, fatherless, motherless, single mothers and fathers. Not only for our church, but for our entire universe. Pray for the homeless.

My Daily Thoughts:

_____

_____

Day 19 *Daily Scripture and Prayer*

Matthew 9:36 -38 - Pray that God will put a greater desire on our hearts to reach the lost and broken hearted around us.

My Daily Thoughts:

_____

_____

_____

Day 20 *Daily Scripture and Prayer*

Micah 6:8 - Pray for our local, state, and nation government leaders, that they would seek God's help as they lead our Nation.

My Daily Thoughts:

_____

_____

_____

Day 21 *Daily Scripture and Prayer*

Psalms 51:14 -15 - Thank the Lord for your salvation; praise Him as we give him honor and praise for the forgiveness of our sins.

My Daily Thoughts:

_____

_____

_____

Recommended Bible app for Bible reading and audio listening: Bible Gateway

CHAPTER 3

Helpful Tips to Stay Focus, Your Purpose and Passion

"8 But Daniel resolved not to defile himself with the royal food and wine, and he asked the chief official for permission not to defile himself this way. 9 Now God has caused the official to favor and compassion to Daniel" *(Daniel 1:8-9, NIV).*

God will be moving in His own way during your fast. Have high expectations that it will be on your behalf. Some people will see changes right away, while others are in incubation and preparing to receive their answer from God. When that incubation period is over, the great work of God is evidence. Expect to build a closer relationship with God and embrace the relationship to be clear on your directions from Him.

When you fast, your body detoxifies, eliminating toxins from the liver, kidney, pancreas, and other organs. If you have never been on a fast before, expect to have some withdrawals. If you drink caffeinated coffee or other beverages daily, or eat sweets (refined sugar), this may cause the withdrawals because you are no longer eating foods or drinking beverages that is toxic to the body. Everybody can benefit from a fast. What other way then to do the *21 –Day Daniel Fast* as you learn how to detox and cleanse the body while praying, submitting to God's will and giving up the foods you like?

Drink plenty of water or lemon water, at least to prepare to hydrate the body to avoid headaches and irritability for any withdrawal symptoms before starting the fast. I prefer drinking hot lemon or zesty lemon water because it quickly detoxes the body and keeps your hunger at bay. The withdrawal symptoms that you will probably experience includes severe to moderate headaches, nausea, insomnia, and irritability. Symptoms will disappear within a few days. Hunger pains are very common when on a fast, so take deep breaths, drink more water for hydration, ease your mind with positive thoughts, and pray often. The fast will enrich your faith, spiritual growth, life's purpose and passion.

Staying focus on God, listening to Him speak to you, and having a positive environment as you fast, will bring unforeseen blessings. Follow Jesus' when you fast. Ask yourself, "What Would Jesus Do While Fasting?". Recall when Jesus was tempted by the devil while fasting 40 days and 40 nights? Let's read the scripture on how Jesus was tempted during His fast. I am hoping this will encourage you to stick with the plan.

> **1** "Then Jesus was led by the Spirit into the wilderness to be tempted by the devil. **2** After fasting forty days and forty nights, he was hungry. **3** The tempter came to him and said, "If you are the Son of God, tell these stones to become bread." **4** Jesus answered, "It is written: 'Man shall not live on bread

alone, but on every word, that comes from the mouth of God."**5** Then the devil took him to the holy city and had him stand on the highest point of the temple. **6** "If you are the Son of God," he said, "throw yourself down. For it is written: "He will command his angels concerning you, and they will lift you up in their hands, so that you will not strike your foot against a stone."

7 Jesus answered him, "It is also written: 'Do not put the Lord your God to the test." **8** Again, the devil took him to a very high mountain and showed him all the kingdoms of the world and their splendor. **9** "All this I will give you," he said, "if you will bow down and worship me."**10** Jesus said to him, "Away from me, Satan! For it is written: 'Worship the Lord your God, and serve him only."

> **11** Then the devil left him, and angels
> came and attended him" *(Matthew 4-1-11*
> *NIV).*

Full-fill and complete the mission of fasting. Know your purpose and passion. There is much more in store for you for being obedient to God's will.

Here are A Heathier You Daniel Fast Tips to Keep You Focus:

AHYDF Tip1: Pray and meditate to ask for strength and direction on the fast throughout the day.

AHYDF Tip 2: Gather with your small group or family for prayer/devotion and bible study.

AHYDF Tip 3: Drink a healthy smoothie to replace a meal, herbal tea, infused water or eat one handful of unsalted nuts.

AHYDF Tip 4: Read your daily scripture and write your daily thoughts down as you pray to God, listen to praise and worship songs, tune into the Christian Channel TV Network or use Bible Gateway to absorb the word. Start or join a small group with people in your church who are on the *21 Day Daniel Fast*. Devotional time with God is an awesome way to fellowship with Him.

AHYDF Tip 5: Make a vision board of your daily walk with God and post things He allows you to see as you pray.

AHYDF Tip 6: Consider doing some moderate exercises.

AHYDF Tip 7: Seek God's face with an open heart and mind daily.

AHYDF Tip 8: Get plenty of rest.

Here are some "A Healthier You Purpose and Passion" Tips

AHYPP 1: Ask God to show you your purpose.

AHYPP 2: Seek likeminded people who have a similar purpose and passion. But most importantly of God's will.

AHYPP 3: Make every day count as your purpose-driven life matures during and after the fast. Always embrace your passion that God has given you. Move toward your life journey goals. Remember God has prepared the way. *AHYPP 4:* Use **S.M.A.R.T.** Goals to enhance your purpose. Submit to the will of God so that He will help you to determine your destiny. Write down how you can address these goals as you complete the *21- Day Daniel Fast*.

AHYPP 5: Use the Bible to find your answers. Know that God will help you as you submit to His purpose for you *(See the table on page 34).*

- S – Specific
- M – Measurable
- A – Attainable
- R – Realistic
- T – Timely

S.M.A. R. T. Goals Chart

Write your S.M.A. R. T. Goals. Pray over them and wait for an answer from God. Make copies of this table for family and friends to complete.

S	
M	
A	
R	
T	

CHAPTER 4

Keeping the Body Functioning During the Fast

When there is a change in your eating habit whether good or bad, your body function changes in how it eliminates bodily fluids. You may feel this is not important because it is a fast, but releasing bowels at least 2-3 times a day and urine that forms a pale yellow to clear indicates that you are hydrated. The body should consist of these healthy functions even if you are not on a fast. You must maintain proper function of your bodies organs when you are fasting too. Especially the liver and the kidneys. Drink 8 glasses or more water every day and eat the suggested foods that will produce the fiber needed for proper elimination of toxins. If you don't like plain water add a ½ squeezed lemon or drink infused water *(Infused water with fruit for 12 to 24 hours for more enhanced flavor)*.

Eliminating Toxins Through Bowel

Eliminating your bowels is important during the fast. Constipation can be a problem. If you are not able to have a bowel movement on the fast, you should drink more water, as well as hot lemon water before and after meals, drink herbal decaffeinated tea (e.g. Smoothe Move, or Hyleys Colon Cleanse Tea) or buy Mag 07 at your local Vitamin Shoppe. We are supposed to eliminate waste at least 2-3 times a day. However, if you drink the tea, drink plenty of water for complete flushing of the bowels.

Balancing Your Body to Food

Food is essential for nourishment of your body. The *21 – Day Daniel Fast* is not a diet, so don't starve if you are not use to fasting. During the fast, you want to adjust your body to foods that you are eating and maintain the purpose of why you are doing the fast. The *21 – Day Daniel Fast* is not easy for those who don't know how to prep their foods for 21 – days. Meal recipes in this book are designed for 2 – day servings and sometimes 3. Servings also depends on the number of people in your family. Since the book consists of breakfast, lunch, and dinner recipes, I suggest you prep for 3 meals a day, include your snacks, desserts, 100 % unsweetened juices and your water. Early morning drink warm or hot lemon (with sliced lemons) or zesty lemon water. Drink at least ½ the body weight in ounces of water daily.

Consider meal replacements with smoothies, it would be sufficient for balancing the body with your food intake. With smoothies you can include snacks and water. Incorporate a moderate cleanse fast: 2 smoothies, sensible meal, 3 snacks, and water or a full cleanse fast: 3 smoothies, 3 snacks, and water. You will still receive the vitamins and antioxidants you need to provide fueling energy throughout the day.

CHAPTER 5

Foods to Eat and Foods to Avoid

4 Jesus answered, "It is written: 'Man shall not live on bread alone, but on every word, that comes from the mouth of God." (Matthew 4:4 NIV).

You are about to embark on a new you and this is only the beginning. As you choose your meals, snacks, and desserts, keep in mind the meaning of the Daniel Fast. Don't over eat just because you are hungry. If you or someone in your family is allergic to any of the foods found in any of the recipes, feel free to make any adjustments to the recipes. Be in prayer for all things that you want God to do for your life, including eating foods that will make you healthy.

Carefully review the charts on the next few pages, make your grocery list, and go shopping for the recipes you would like to try for the next 21-days (3 weeks). Make sure you read labels on all food products. Just because the non-brand food item is cheap, does not mean that it contains the same ingredient as the brand name food item. Additives and preservatives are what you should watch for. If it is found in the ***ingredient*** that make-up the food item, it is in the food (e.g. sugar corn syrup or high fructose, MSG, trans-fat, common food dyes, sodium sulfite, etc.).

Organic foods are the best foods to buy. Why buy organic? Organic foods are regulated by the federal government, it is healthier and safe. You can avoid food allergies, an unhealthy gut, and chronic illnesses. But if you are like me, on a budget, buy the fresh or frozen fruit and vegetables. Non-organic foods are treated with herbicides and pesticides which often contributes to hormonal changes in the body, inflammation, obesity, disorders, and diseases such as cancer, arthritis, hypertension (high blood pressure), fibromyalgia, Lupus, allergies, gout, skin disorders (e.g. acne, dry, oily, scaly), colds, flu, bronchitis, etc. However, when you buy non-organic foods, wash the food thoroughly with apple cider or white vinegar and water. I usually allow my raw fruit to soak for 2-5 minutes in the vinegar and water, pat dry before eating or adding the fruit to my smoothies. Most of the fruit that I buy is frozen which is best for making great tasting smoothies.

Pre-packaged vegetables in the bags are pre-washed according to the imprint on the bad. I rinse the vegetables again before using. I suggest when buying bagged fresh vegetables, buy zip lock bags to freeze them. The vegetables last longer in the freezer than in the refrigerator.

Prepping your smoothies for 5 days will make it easier if you go to work early morning. Use small zip lock bags and place all ingredients in the bag. Start with your fruit first and then greens. Pour your prep smoothie in your blender and be on your way. Don't forget to date your zip lock bags too.

Foods to Eat Chart

Whole Grains	Brown Rice, Barley, Oat, Quinoa
Legumes	Dried Beans, Mix Beans, Pinto Beans, Split Peas, Lentils, Black Beans, Black Eyed Peas, Navy Beans, Cannellini Beans
Fruit	Apples, Apricots, Bananas, Blackberries, Blueberries, Boysenberries, Cantaloupe, Cherries, Cranberries, Figs, Grapefruit, Grapes, Guava, Honeydew, Melon, Kiwi, Lemons. Limes, Mangos, Majool Dates, Nectarines, Papayas, Peaches, Pears, Pineapples, Plums, Prunes, Raisins, Raspberries, Strawberries, Tomatoes, Tangelos Tangerines, Unsweetened Coconut Flakes, Watermelon, **All-Natural Frozen Fruit**
Vegetables	Artichokes, Asparagus, Beets, Broccoli, Brussels Sprouts, Cabbage, Carrots, Cauliflower, Celery, Chili Pepper, Collard Greens, Corn, Cucumbers, Eggplant, Garlic, Green Peppers, Ginger Root, Kale, Leeks, Lettuce, Mushrooms, Mustard Greens, Okra, Onions, Orange Peppers, Parsley, Potatoes, Radishes, Rutabagas, Scallions, Spinach, Sprouts, Squashes, Sweet Potatoes, Red Peppers, Turnips, Watercress, Yams, Yellow Peppers, Zucchini
Oils	Extra Virgin, Unrefined Coconut, Grapeseed, Sesame
Nuts/Seeds	Cashews, Chia Seed, Flaxseeds, Mixed Nuts,

(Unsalted & Unflavored)	Peanuts, Pecan, Sunflower, Walnuts
Liquids	Apple Cider Vinegar, Decaffeinated Herbal Tea 100 % Fruit Juice, 100 % Vegetable Juices, Unsweetened Coconut/Almond Milk, Coconut Water, Water (Spring, Alkaline, or Purified),
Seasonings	All Spice, Almond Flour, Parsley, Basil, Bay Leaves, Black Pepper, Cayenne Pepper, Cajun Natural, Chili Powder, Cinnamon, Cocoa Powder Coconut Flour, Coconut Sugar, Stevia, Corn Starch, Cumin, Garlic Powder, Nutmeg, Onion Powder, Organic Thyme, Turmeric, 100 % Pure Himalayan Ancient Pink Sea Salt, Rice Vinegar, Salt Free Seasoning Sea Salt, Turmeric, Wheat Flour, White Pepper

The most importance of the fast is to pray and meditate on God's word. Don't worry about the food you will eat. The Lord will provide you with the right substance.

Foods to Avoid Chart

It will be difficult to avoid certain foods during the fast. Your hunger pains will be very real. To complete the fast and see the changes that God will bring into your life, you must exclude these foods:

• All Meats • Fish • White rice, • Fried foods • Dairy products • Eggs • Caffeine • Alcohol • Breads	• Chips • Crackers • White flour and all products using it • Margarine & shortening, high fat products. • Carbonated beverages • Foods with preservatives/additives, • Refined sugar, corn syrup, sugar substitutes

Additives and Preservatives to Avoid Chart

Sugar
High Fructose (Corn Syrup)
Food Dyes (e.g. Blue #1 &2, Red #3, Red#40, Yellow #6 and Yellow Tartrazine
Sodium Sulfite
Butylated Hydroxyanisole (BHA) and Butylate Hydroxytoluene (BHT)
Sulfur Dioxide
Potassium Bromate
Monosodium Glutamate (MSG)
Trans-fat

Be Aware:

Be careful about additives and preservatives. Most non-brand products have added to the ingredients to give you the satisfying taste of the food. The additives and preservatives can cause major health problems in the future. Choose wisely and stick with the plan.

CHAPTER 6

What's for Breakfast Recipes?

You have recipes below to determine what you want for breakfast. Choose your breakfast menu as you start day 1 on the Daniel Fast.

Grits and Potatoes

Cook grits until done add a small amount of sea salt and liquid popcorn butter flavor.

Stove Top White Potatoes

peel potatoes (dice or slice)

3 chopped scallions

½ chopped onions

1 tsp black pepper

1 tsp sea salt

1 tsp garlic powder

1 tsp onion powder

1 tsp parsley or fresh parsley

2 tbsps. extra virgin olive or grape seed oil

Directions:

Add 1 tbsp. oil to the mixture and stir to blend all ingredients in a large bowl.
Pour 1 tbsp. olive or grape seed oil into a skillet. Stir potatoes occasionally until brown.

Oatmeal Apple Raisin Bake (Morning or Evening Treat)

1 cup plain oatmeal

½ cup 100% unsweetened apple juice or orange juice

2 sliced granny apples or McIntosh apples

2 tbsps. grapeseed oil

1 to 2 tsps. cinnamon

½ cup raisins

½ cup of walnuts or pecans

2 tsps. raw or unfiltered date honey

¼ cup of liquid flavor popcorn oil or unrefined coconut oil

Directions:

Add all ingredients in a bowl. Place mixed ingredients in a baking dish. Pour oil with grapeseed or olive oil. Bake at 350 until golden brown. Drizzle your treat with orange juice and oil.

Pineapple Muffins

1 cup rolled oats

1 cup wheat flour

½ cup diced pineapples

¼ cup chopped pecans or walnuts

½ cup raisins

¼ cup date honey

¼ cup flaxseed milled

2 tsps. unsweetened coconut flakes

2 tsps. grated orange zest

¼ teaspoon ground ginger

Potato Cabbage

5 potatoes cut in cubes

½ cabbage

4 carrots shredded or sliced

1 onion sliced

1 tsp. ground black pepper

1 teaspoon sea salt

½ cup olive oil

½ tsp. ground cumin

¼ tsp. ground turmeric

Directions:

Heat olive oil in a skillet over medium heat. Cook the carrots and onion in the oil for about 5 minutes. Stir in the salt, pepper, cumin, turmeric, and cabbage and cook another 15 to 20 minutes. Add the potatoes; cover. Reduce heat to medium-low and cook until potatoes are soft, 20 to 30 minutes.

Tofu Egg Scrambler

1 box firm tofu

1 tomato diced

¼ cup onions diced

1 tomato diced

2 tbsps. olive oil

½ onion diced

1 red pepper diced

2 green onions chopped

1 tbsp. fresh cilantro minced

1 clove garlic minced

Add salt and pepper to taste

Tomato pasted if desired

Directions:

Pat tofu dry and roll in a clean, absorbent towel with something heavy on top, such as a cast iron skillet, for 15 minutes. Set aside. Prep veggies and warm a large skillet over medium heat. Once hot, add 1-2 tbsp. olive oil and the onion and red pepper. Season with a pinch each salt and pepper and stir. Cook until softened - about 5 minutes. In the meantime, unwrap tofu and use a fork to crumble into bite-sized pieces.

Use a spatula to move the veggies to one side of the pan and add tofu. Stir immediately, evenly distributing the sauce. Cook for another 5-7 minutes until tofu is slightly browned. Serve immediately with the breakfast potatoes. Add more flavor with salsa.

Breakfast Shake or Any Time Shake

Almond Chocolate Peanut Butter

1 cup unsweetened almond or coconut milk (cold)

1 ripe banana

2 tbsps. unsweetened peanut butter

1 tsp. unsweetened cocoa powder Toll House

1/2 cup ice

Strawberry Shake

1 cup unsweetened coconut milk (cold)

1 ½ cup frozen strawberries

2 packets Stevia

CHAPTER 7

Lunch and Dinner is Served Recipes

Roasted Red Pepper Spaghetti w/Sauce

1 box whole grain spaghetti

3 Roma tomatoes diced

1 large can tomato paste (No salt) (Optional)

½ cup Hunt's tomato sauce (No salt)

1 red bell pepper diced

1 cup fresh parsley or 2 tbsp. parsley flakes

½ diced onions

5 chopped scallions

2 basil leaves or 1 tsp. chopped basil leaves

1 tsp. oregano

1 10 oz. can mushroom

4 tbsps. olive oil or grape seed oil

1/8 tsp. white pepper

1 tsp. black pepper

2 tsps. garlic powder

1 tbsp. minced garlic

2 tsp. onion powder

1 tsp sea salt

Directions:

Boil the spaghetti with sea salt or garlic powder until done. Toss red peppers and tomatoes in 1 tsp sea salt and 1 tbsp. of oil. On a cooking tray roast diced tomatoes and red peppers for 10 minutes. In a large sauce pan add 3 tablespoons of olive or grape seed oil. Stir onions scallions, minced garlic, and seasonings for 5-8 minutes. Add the mushrooms, parsley and tomato sauce to the sauce pan and simmer for 15-20 minutes. Serve the sauce over the spaghetti.

Black Bean Vegan Patties

1 (15oz) can black beans

1 ½ cup brown rice

4 scallions chopped

½ fresh parsley chopped

½ onion chopped

2 tbsps. olive oil

1 tsp. chili powder

1 tsp. cumin

2 tbsps. corn starch

2 tsps. garlic powder

2 tsps. onion powder

1 tsp. sea salt

1tsp. black pepper

Directions:

Boil brown rice until fluffy and set aside. Drain and rinse black beans. Pat dry, sprinkle garlic powder over beans, and spread beans on parchment paper. Place in oven at 350 for 5-8 minutes or until slightly plump or toasted. Let the beans cool for 3 minutes. If you have food processor of vegetable chopper, grind the black beans until it is grounded. Put ground beans in a bowl. Add seasonings and parsley. In a sauce pan, cook chopped onions, and scallions in olive oil for 5 minutes. Add ½ cup of rice in the sauce pan and stir for 3 minutes. Add more olive oil to keep the mixture from sticking. Add the onions, scallions, and rice mix to the grounded beans and stir. Add the cup of rice and the cornstarch and fold it into the grounded beans. Divide the mixture to make 8 patties. In a skillet, heat 2 tbsps. of olive oil on low heat. Cook patties for 3-4 minutes. Serve hot! (Add green bell peppers for more flavor)

Potato Corn Soup

6-8 peeled and diced potatoes

1 bag frozen corn

1 peeled chopped onion

5 chopped scallions

6 stalks celery diced

1 ½ cup organic vegetable broth

6 cups water

2 cups coconut milk

1 tbsp. olive, coconut or grapeseed oil

1 tsp. popcorn flavor oil (Optional)

2 tsps. garlic powder

2 tsps. onion powder

1 tsp. sea salt

1tsp. black pepper

¼ tsp. white pepper

Directions:

Boil potatoes in 6 cups of water until slightly soft. Drain water and sit the potatoes aside. Sauté celery, onions, and scallions in 1 tbsp. olive oil. In a separate boiler add 2 tbsp. of popcorn flavor ½ tsp. garlic powder and corn. Sauté for 10 minutes. Add sautéed celery, onions, and scallions, corn, coconut milk, and organic vegetable broth to the potatoes. If the soup is to thick, add a little water. Simmer for 10 minutes. You can cook this in a slow cooker also.

Stir Fry Veggie and Pasta

1 bag veggie spirals pasta

2 tbsps. olive or grape seed oil

1 bag frozen broccoli

1 small bag frozen corn

1 green and red Pepper

2 chopped scallions

1 can string beans (Drained)

1 tsp black pepper

½ tsp sea salt

1 tsp. garlic powder

½ parsley flakes

1 tsp. onion powder.

1 can peas and carrots (Drained)

½ fresh sliced pineapples

2 mandarin oranges or tangerines

Directions:

Boil Veggie spirals in a pot. Use a large skillet to stir fry your veggies add, olive or grapeseed oil, add seasonings and stir for 10 minutes. Add fresh sliced pineapples and mandarin oranges or tangerines. Squeeze three to four of the mandarin oranges or tangerines into the stir fry and cook for 5 more minutes.

Chili Bean

1 bag kidney beans

4 diced scallions

2 tbsps. extra virgin olive Oil

1 bell pepper

1 garlic clove

1 chopped onion

1 tbsp. parsley

2 tsps. chili powder

1 pack McCormick chili seasoning

1 can peeled, chopped tomatoes or fresh tomatoes

1 can tomato paste

Directions:

Soak kidney beans overnight. Place kidney beans in a crock pot or boil in a pot for 1 ½ hour. Heat oil in a saucepan to cook scallions, onions, pepper, garlic cloves and tomatoes until tender. Add seasoning ingredients and cook for an additional hour.

Red or White Baked Potatoes

10 -15 diced potatoes with skin

3 scallions

½ chopped onions

1 red bell pepper

2 tbsps. olive oil or grape seed oil

¼ tsp. cayenne pepper

1 tsp. black pepper

1 tsp. sea salt

1 ½ tsp. garlic powder

1 tsp parsley flakes

1 ½ tsp. onion powder

Directions:

Put olive oil or grapeseed oil in a mixing bowl add seasonings and stir. Pour sliced or diced potatoes with skin and mix with oil and seasoning. Spread the mixture on parchment paper and bake in the oven at 350 for 25 minutes until golden brown. *Optional recipe: Bake sliced potatoes with skin without the red peppers, scallions, and onions*

Lima Beans and Black Eye Peas (Stir Fry and Boil)

1 bag frozen lima beans

1 bag frozen black eye peas

3-4 tsp. extra virgin olive or grapeseed oil

1tsp. garlic powder

1 tsp. onion powder

¾ tsp. black pepper

Directions:

Heat the oil slightly in a pot and add all seasonings. Add the frozen lima beans and black eye peas to the oil and seasoning. Stir continuously for 15 -20 minutes to avoid sticking. Add water and boil for 25-30 more minutes or until beans are tender.

Stir Fry Collard Greens

1-2 bags frozen greens

3-4 tbsps. extra virgin olive or grape seed oil

½ green bell pepper (sliced strips)

½ red bell pepper (sliced strips)

3-4 scallions chopped

1 tsp. garlic powder

2 tsp. minced garlic

1 tsp. onion powder

½ bag okra (Optional)

Directions:

In a large skillet add oil of choice. Stir fry the green, red bell peppers, and scallions. Add seasonings. Add greens to the mixture and stir fry for 20 minutes add more seasoning if desired. Add the okra. Cook until done.

Stir Fry Kale Collard Greens

1 bag frozen fresh greens

1 bag frozen or fresh kale

3-4 tbsps. extra virgin olive or grape seed oil

3-4 scallions chopped

1 tsp. garlic powder

2 tsp. minced garlic

1 tsp. onion powder

Directions:

In a large skillet add oil of choice and stir fry scallions. Add seasonings. Add greens to the mixture and stir fry for 20 minutes add more seasoning if desired. Cook until done.

Pasta Spinach Salad

1 bag whole wheat penne pasta

1 cup chopped spinach

1 red bell pepper (sliced trips)

1 pack cherry tomatoes

1 whole garlic clove

2 tsps. garlic powder

2 tsps. onion powder

1 tsp. sea salt

2 tbsp. olive or grapeseed oil

Directions:

Boil penne pasta until tender and drain water. Coat whole garlic clove with olive oil and close in aluminum foil bake in the oven for 10 -15 minutes. Peel off skin and mince in a small bowl. Put plum tomatoes and red bell peppers on a cook sheet and sprinkled with sea salt. Place in oven until plum tomatoes are bursting open. In a large bowl stir in seasonings, spinach, tomatoes, and red bell peppers. Stir in cooked pasta and serve hot or cold.

Sautéed Spinach w/Roma Tomatoes

2 cups spinach

¼ tsp. sea salt

1 tsp. garlic powder

1 tsp. onion powder

1 tbsp. olive or grapeseed oil

½ tsp. flake parsley or ¼ chopped fresh parsley

1 sliced Roma tomato

Directions:

Sautéed spinach in olive oil or grape seed oil. Add seasonings and heat for 10-15 minutes. Sautéed Roma tomato the same as the spinach and add parsley. Add tomatoes to the spinach and serve

Black Bean Quesadillas

1 can black beans (drained/rinsed)

¾ cup diced tomatoes

pinch cayenne pepper

glove garlic

1tsp. ground cumin

8 tsp. chili powder

8 whole grains tortillas

Directions:

Blend black beans, 3/4 cup tomatoes, and garlic in a food processor until smooth; add nutritional yeast, cumin, chili powder, salt, and cayenne pepper flakes and blend again. Add bean mixture to a bowl. Stir black beans and 1/4 cup tomatoes into bean mixture. Heat olive oil in a skillet over medium-high heat.

Place a tortilla in the hot oil. Spread about 1/4 cup filling onto the tortilla. Place another tortilla on top of filling; cook until filling is warmed, about 10 minutes. ½ tsp. olive oil on top tortilla and flip quesadilla to cook the second side until lightly browned, 3 to 5 minutes. Repeat with remaining tortillas and filling.

Sweet Potato Mash

4 sweet potatoes

½ cup unsweetened coconut milk

2 tbsps. popcorn flavor oil or vegan butter

1 tsp. cinnamon

Directions:

Boiled sweet potatoes in a large pot until soften. Peel skin from the potatoes and place in a bowl. Add the coconut milk, cinnamon, and popcorn flavor. Whipped with a blender until ingredients are mixed.

Apple Cinnamon Brown Rice

¾ cup uncooked brown rice

1 ½ cups unsweetened apple juice

1 apple cored and chopped

1/3 cup raisins

½ tsp. cinnamon

¼ tsp. sea salt

¼ cup chopped fresh parsley

Directions:

In a saucepan, combine rice, apple juice, chopped apple, and raisins. Season with cinnamon and salt. Bring to a boil, reduce heat to low, and cover for about 17 minutes. When cooking with brown rice it takes 25-30 minutes; if not, cook for 3 more minutes. Mix in fresh parsley. Serve immediately.

Cabbage Soup

5 carrots sliced

1 onion chopped

2 whole peeled tomatoes

1 large cabbage chopped

1 (15 ounce) green beans, drained

½ quart tomato juice

1 green bell pepper diced

5 stalks celery chopped

1 ½ cup vegetable broth

1 tsp. garlic powder

1 tsp. onion powder

¼ tsp. sea salt

Directions:

Place carrots, onions, tomatoes (boil tomatoes until soften), cabbage, green beans, peppers, and celery in a large pot. Add seasonings, tomato juice, beef broth, and enough water to cover vegetables. Cook vegetables on low heat until tender. May be stored in the refrigerator for several days.

Mixed Bean Soup

1 cup brown rice

1 (16oz) bag mixed beans (rinsed and soaked for 30 minutes)

1(16oz) frozen spinach

1 cup shredded carrots

3 cups water

2 cups organic vegetable broth

2 tbsps. virgin olive oil

1 chopped onions

1 red bell pepper (chopped)

1 green bell pepper (chopped)

½ cup scallions (chopped)

¼ cup parsley

4 celery stalks (chopped)

2 tbsps. minced garlic

1 tsp. garlic powder

1 tsp. onion powder

½ tsp thyme

1 tsp. black pepper

½ tsp. white pepper

1 pinch cayenne pepper

½ tsp. sea salt

Directions:

Add beans, vegetables, and seasoning to water in a crock pot. Allow the bean and vegetables, except for the onion to cook for 6 ½ hours. Drain 1 cup of water from the beans and vegetables. Add olive oil to a saucepan on low heat add frozen spinach and onions. Season to taste use garlic and onion powder and stir fry. Add vegetable broth parsley and stir for 5 minutes. Add mixture to the beans and vegetables and cook for 2 more hours. Serve with cooked brown rice. Soup last for 2 -3 days.

Sweet Potato Vegetable Soup

1 medium sweet potato, peeled and cut into 1" cubes

3 carrots, peeled and sliced

1 stalk celery, diced

1 small yellow onion, diced

1 clove garlic, minced

Pinch of Kosher or sea salt, to taste

1/2 teaspoon black pepper

1/8 teaspoon allspice

1 teaspoon paprika

1 bay leaf

2 (15 ounce) cans kidney beans, drained and rinsed
(optional, black or navy beans)

4 cups vegetable broth, low-sodium

1 (14.5 oz.) can diced tomatoes (no salt added),

4 cups baby spinach, loosely packed

1 tablespoon plus 1 teaspoon extra-virgin olive oil,
optional, for serving (1/2 teaspoon per serving)

Directions:

Add all ingredients, except spinach and olive oil, to the slow cooker. Cover and cook on low 6 to 8 hours, or until the vegetables are tender. Add spinach, stir and continue cooking just until wilted, approximately 5 minutes. Serve and enjoy!

Tip: Try a thicker soup, after 5 hours of cooking, by removing 1 cup of soup, along with ingredients, mash ingredients with a fork, return to the slow cooker, stir and continue cooking 1 to 3 hours. When serving, drizzle a little (optional) olive oil over each bowl of soup.

Veggie Wrap

8 wheat wraps or wraps with flaxseed and olive oil or garden spinach herb wraps (Can be purchased at Walmart)
1 bag mixed peppers and onions
or 1 red, yellow, and, green pepper, onion (sliced strips)
1 cup shredded lettuce or spinach
1 chopped tomato

1 tsp. olive oil or grapeseed oil

½ tsp. garlic powder

½ tsp onion powder

1 pinch sea salt

1 pinch pepper

1 tsp. Bragg's apple cider vinegar (Optional)

Directions:

Add mixed peppers and onions to a saucepan with heated olive oil. Add seasonings and stir fry vegetables until tender or roast vegetables in oven. Heat tortillas in the stove or microwave for 15 seconds. Place shredded lettuce or spinach to the heated tortilla. Add vegetables, sea salt, pepper, and drizzle apple cider vinegar.

Bonus Lunch and Dinner Is Served Recipes

Delicious Roasted Veggie Pizza with Toppings

1 green bell pepper (sliced into strips)

5 red sweet cherry peppers (sliced) or 1 red bell pepper

1 cup packed spinach (cut)

½ small onion (sliced into strips)

1-10 oz. can mushroom (drained)

1-10 oz. can black olives (drained)

1 tsp sea salt

2 tbsps. extra virgin olive oil

Optional Toppings

"Cashew Mozzarella" *(See directions below Pizza Sauce)*

½ sliced Roma tomato

1 tsp. crushed red peppers

Directions:

Pre-heat oven 350

Use a cookie sheet and cover with parchment paper. Put veggies in a bowl. Add and toss extra virgin olive oil and sea salt to cover all veggies. Spread veggies on the parchment paper and roast for 10-15 minutes.

Pizza Sauce

3-4 Roma Tomatoes (thinly sliced)

1 – can or jarred tomato paste or sauce (unsalted)

2 basil leaves or 1 tsp. chopped basil leaves

1 tsp. oregano

1 tsp. fresh squeezed lemon

½ tbsp. olive oil or grape seed oil

1 tsp. black pepper

2 tsps. garlic powder

2 tsp. onion powder

1 tsp sea salt

Directions:

Use a blender or a food processor. Add ingredients to the blender or processor and extract until mixture is smooth.

Directions for "Cashew Mozzarella" *(Inspired by Nutribullet Life Changing Recipes)*

Pre-heat Broiler

Use a blender or a food processor. Add ingredients to the blender or processor and extract
for 50 second increments, pausing for 30 seconds in between each, until mixture is smooth. Spoon several dollops of cashew cheese on top to shape like mozzarella rounds. Top with tomato slices and basil leaves and heat under broiler for 5 minutes until basils shrivel and other toppings are warm. Watch closely the toppings can quickly burn.

Pizza Crust *(Inspired by Nutribullet Life Changing Recipes)*

1 ½ cups quinoa, soaked and drained
½ cup filtered water

1 tsp. sea salt

3 Tbsp. olive or cold pressed virgin coconut oil divided into two 1 ½ Tbsp. portions

Directions:

Preheat oven to 450 degrees

In a blender or food processor, soak quinoa, water, and salt and extract in the blender or processor until combined. Add more water if necessary. Your mixture should resemble pancake batter.

Coat the base and sides of two 8-inch cake pans with divided olive or coconut oil, and heat in the oven until the oil starts to bubble. Remove from the oven and pour half of the crust batter into each pan. Bake for 20 minutes, then flip the crusts and bake an additional 5-8 minutes. Spread pizza sauce on the quinoa crust and toppings. Bake for 5 minutes. Don't over bake.

Black Bean Dip

2 cans organic bean (drained and rinsed)

or 3 cups cooked black beans

½ onion (chopped)

1 clove garlic, minced

1 small jalapeno pepper (de-seeded and diced)

4- cherry tomatoes, rinsed

¼ red bell pepper (chopped)

1 squeezed lime juice

¼ tsp. tsp ground cumin

¼ tsp chili powder

Sea salt and pep

per to taste

Directions:

Add all ingredients to your blender, food processor to
extract, or a bowl to stir and blend. Scrape the sides from

what you are using to blend the ingredients until ingredients form a thick paste. Eat with corn or wheat tortillas.

CHAPTER 8

21-Days of Healthy Smoothies

Tips for Blending Great Smoothies and Drinking Your Smoothies.

AHYDF Tip 1: Blend your greens first for 30 seconds with a liquid then add your fruit and blend for an additional 30 seconds or until smooth.

AHYDF Tip 2: Chew your smoothies for easy digestion and to fill full

AHYDF Tip 3: Drink smoothies for breakfast, lunch or dinner as a meal replacement.

Frozen Fruit Smoothie

1 cup unsweetened almond milk

1 bag frozen strawberry and mango (Or any frozen fruit combination)

1 ripe banana

1 cup whole or crushed ice

Mango Strawberry Smoothie

2 cups unsweetened coconut milk

1 ½ cup frozen mango

½ cup frozen or fresh strawberries

1 ripe banana

If desired, add ice as you blend for a thicker smoothie

Green Smoothie

1 handful spinach

1 handful kale

1 peeled kiwi

2 stalks celery

4-5 slices cucumber

1 green apple

1 handful frozen green grapes

3-4 slices of fresh ginger root

¼ cup lemon juice

½ cup spring or purified water

Go Green

1 cup spinach

½ ripe banana

1 avocado (peeled and pit removed)

1 tbsp. sunflower seeds

½ cup lemon juice

1 cup unsweetened almond milk

Apple Carrot

2 carrots

2 stalks celery

1 green apple

2 leaves kale

½ cup fresh parsley

Apple Cinnamon Cranberry

3 handful spinach

1 cup water

2 cored green apples

1 cup red seedless grapes or green seedless grapes

1½ cup frozen fresh cranberries (pitted fresh cranberries)

2 celery stalks

1 bunch parsley

1 tsp. cinnamon

1 tsp. fresh turmeric or ground

1 tbsps. grounded flaxseeds

Tropical Mango Banana

1 handful spinach

1 cup coconut water or unsweetened coconut milk

1 tbsp. coconut oil

½ cup frozen mango

1 banana

¼ cup unsweetened pineapple juice

Blueberry Spinach Coconut

1 handful spinach (Optional)

1 tbsp. coconut oil

½ cup frozen blueberries

1 tsp. nuts or seeds (unsalted)

½ cup unsweetened coconut milk

¼ cup rolled oats

Spinach Pineapple

2 handfuls spinach

1 cup frozen pineapple

1 cored pear

1 cup parsley

½ grapefruit peeled

Peachy Grapes

1 ripe peach (Pitted)

1 cup frozen blueberries

½ cup red or green grapes

½ cup prunes

Apple Papaya Smoothie

2 handfuls kale

1 handful spinach

1 cored apple

1-2 cup water

1 cup frozen or fresh papaya

½ cup frozen or fresh strawberries

1 cup frozen or fresh peaches

2 tbsps. flaxseeds (ground or mill)

Tropical Lemon Orange Berry

2 handfuls spinach

1 cups water

1 cup seedless red grapes

1 cup frozen or fresh blueberries

A Healthier You w/Dr. V. Benson
21- Day Daniel Fast Recipes

1 orange peeled and deseeded

1 lemon peeled or ¼ cup lemon juice

1 lime peeled

1 tbsp. flaxseeds (ground or mill)

Spinach Kale Berry Smoothie

1 handful spinach

2 handfuls kale

1 cup water

1 banana peeled

1 bunch parsley

1 ½ cup frozen or fresh blueberries

1 ½ cup frozen or fresh blackberries

1 cup fresh red or black grapes

2 tbsps. flaxseeds (ground or mill)

Banana Pineapple Smoothie

2 handfuls spring mix greens

1 cup water

1 banana peeled

1 cup frozen pineapple chunks

1 cup fresh seedless red grapes

2 celery stalks chopped

2 slices ginger root (washed and skinned) or 1 tsp. ground ginger

2 tbsps. flaxseeds (ground or mill)

Peach Raspberry

1 cup unsweetened almond or coconut milk

1 ½ cup frozen raspberry

1 cup frozen mango

1 cup frozen sliced peaches

Orange Apple Banana

1 cup unsweetened orange juice

½ banana peeled

½ cored apple

1 cup ice

Pineapple Cranberry Kale

1 cup kale

1 cup parsley

1 celery stalk

1 cucumber

1 cup frozen or fresh pineapples

1 cup frozen or fresh cranberries (Pitted)

Banana Strawberry Orange

1 handful spinach

½ cup water

1 banana

1 cup strawberries

1 squeezed orange or ¼ cup unsweetened orange juice

½ cup of walnuts

Berry Mango

1 handful spinach

2 handfuls kale

1 cored apple

1 banana peeled

1 cup mango

1 cup water

Tropical Pineapple Blueberry Lime

1 cup unsweetened coconut milk

1 cup frozen pineapples

1 cup frozen blueberries

½ cup lime (100%) juice

Avocado Blueberry Mango

1 cup unsweetened coconut milk

1 cup frozen or fresh blueberries

1 cup frozen or fresh mango

½ cup almonds

1 tsp. cinnamon

1 handful pecans (Optional)

Bonus Smoothies

Cran-Pomegranate Berry

1 handful kale

1 frozen banana

½ cup frozen mixed berries

1 cup frozen blueberries

½ cup cran-pomegranate (Ocean Spray 100% Juice)

1 tbsp. hemp seed

1 tbsp. grounded flaxseeds

Blueberry Banana

2 handfuls spinach

1 cup water

1 banana

1 cored apple

1 cup frozen chunk pineapples

1 cup frozen blueberries

2 tbsp. grounded flaxseeds

Plum Peach Smoothie

2 handfuls spring mix greens

2 handfuls spinach

1 ½ cup water

1 cored plum

1 cup frozen peaches

1 cup frozen pineapples

2 tbsp. grounded flaxseeds

Citrus Green Smoothie

2 handfuls baby spinach

1 large orange

½ squeezed fresh lemon or lime (1tsp. lemon or lime juice)

1 cup frozen strawberries

Pineapple Peach

3 handfuls spring mix greens

2 handfuls spinach

2 bananas peeled

1 ½ cup water

1 ½ cup frozen pineapple chunk

1 cup frozen peaches

2 tbsp. grounded flaxseeds.

New Tropical Green Smoothie

1 cup unsweetened Tropicana orange juice

2 handfuls baby spinach

1 banana peeled

1 cup frozen pineapples

1 cup frozen strawberries

1/2 cup frozen mangos

1 handful almonds (unsalted)

CHAPTER 9
The Perfect Green Salad and Dressing Recipes

Green Fruit Salad

4-5 cups spring mix & spinach or garden mix greens

1 cup red or green grapes (halved)

8-10 strawberries (sliced)

1- 2 diced apples (place apples in 2 tablespoons of lemon juice until ready to eat salad to keep from browning).

1-2 diced or sliced Roma tomatoes raisins (Optional)

Directions:

Toss in ingredients in a bowl to mix.

Vinaigrette Salad Dressing

½ cup olive oil

½ cup of grape seed Oil

¼ cup of lemon juice or ½ squeezed lemon

1tsp. sea salt

1tsp. black pepper

3- 4 pinches of red pepper or cayenne pepper

3 tsps. garlic powder

1 tsp. onion powder

2 tsps. Mrs. Dash or unsalted seasoning (Dollar Tree).

Directions:

Stir or shake in a bottle or Ziploc bag until mixed.

Green Apple Walnut Salad

1 handful spring mixed power greens

½ cup baby spinach

1 green apple (cored, sliced)

8-10 strawberries (sliced)

1 handful walnuts or pecans (toasted)

Strawberry Salad Dressing

¼ cup olive oil

¼ cup Braggs apple cider vinegar

5 frozen strawberries (pureed)

¼ cup water

½ lemon or 4 tbsps. lemon juice

¼ tsp. sea salt

1 tsp. garlic powder

1 tsp. onion powder

1 tsp. Cajun spice

1 tsp. Cajun spice (McCormick Perfect Pinch)

1 tsp salad supreme (McCormick Perfect Pinch)

Directions:

Blend vegetables and fruit ingredients in a bowl. Toast walnuts or pecans for 3-5 minutes and spread over salad. Puree strawberries with water blend and with other dressing ingredients. Slightly warm the dressing and pour over salad.

Apple Cucumber Salad

1 diced apple

1 diced cucumber

2 tbsps. Braggs Apple Cider Vinegar (ACV)

Directions:

Mixed diced apples and cucumber toss in ACV

Raspberry Salad Dressing

¼ cup olive oil

1 cup raspberry (pureed)

¼ cup Braggs apple cider vinegar

½ lemon or 4 tbsps. lemon juice

¼ tsp. sea salt

1 tsp. garlic powder

1 tsp. onion powder

Directions:

Shake or stir in glass jar with top. Store in the refrigerator until ready to use.

Mandarin Kiwi Spinach Salad w/Orange Poppy Seed Dressing

4-5 spinach

4 cups of Romaine lettuce

4 kiwis

2 mandarins peeled and separated

¼ cup sliced red onions

¼ raisins (Optional)

Directions:

Mix ingredients in a large bowl

Orange Poppy Seed Salad Dressing

¼ cup extra virgin olive or grapeseed oil

2 tsps. fresh lemon or lemon juice

¼ cup orange juice

1/8 tsp dry mustard

1/8 tsp. sea salt

¼ tsp. poppy seeds

Directions:

Place in a glass jar with top and the refrigerator until ready to use.

Black Corn Salad

4 cups spinach

1 ½ cup corn

½ cup cherry tomatoes sliced in halves

2 cans (15 ounces) black beans drained

4 scallions chopped

1 avocado peeled and diced

1 red bell pepper

1 clove, minced

½ cup cilantro (Optional)

Directions:

In a large bowl, combine beans, corn, avocado, bell pepper, tomatoes, scallions, onions, and cilantro. Shake lime dressing, and pour it over the salad. Stir salad to coat vegetables and beans with dressing, and serve.

Lime Salad Dressing

1/3 cup lime juice
½ cup olive oil
1clove garlic minced
1/8 tsp. cayenne
¼ tsp. sea salt

Directions:

Place lime juice, olive oil, garlic, salt, and cayenne pepper in a small jar. Cover with lid, and shake until ingredients are well mixed.

CHAPTER 10

Snacks and Desserts

Apple Butter Drizzle

1 sliced green apple cored

2 tbsps. unsweetened peanut butter or almond butter

1 tsp. apple cider vinegar or lemon juice

Directions:

Toss apples in apple cider vinegar or lemon juice. Pour off apple cider vinegar or lemon juice. Melt butter of choice and drizzle over apples.

Creamy Pineapple Delight Ice Cream

1 cup almond or coconut milk (Unsweetened)

1 cup frozen or fresh pineapples

1tsp. vanilla extract (without alcohol content) or fresh vanilla bean plant

½ cup ice

Directions:

Add all ingredients in the blender and serve cold.

Tortillas and Salsa

1 can chopped tomatoes or 3 fresh chopped tomatoes

½ cup chopped green peppers

1 cup diced onions

¼ cup minced or fresh cilantro

2 tsps. lime juice

4 tsps. chopped jalapeno (include seeds)

½ tsp. ground cumin

½ tsp. kosher salt

½ tsp. ground black pepper

1 bag tortillas

Directions:

Stir the tomatoes, green bell pepper, onion, cilantro, lime juice, jalapeno pepper, cumin, salt, and pepper in a bowl. Serve with tortillas.

Tortillas and Mango Salsa

1 ripe mango (peeled, pitted)

½ cucumber

1 jalapeno pepper (halved, seeds removed)

¼ avocado

¼ cup fresh lime juice

½ tsp dried cumin

5 sprigs fresh cilantro (stems removed)

Directions:

Add ingredients to a blender or food processor or stir in bowl until smoothie and creamy. Serve with tortillas

Popping Popcorn

½ cup of popcorn Kernels

1 tbsp. coconut oil

¼ tsp. sea salt (Optional)

¼ tsp. garlic powder

¼ tsp onion powder

1 tsp. paprika

1 tsp lemon pepper

¼ tsp cayenne pepper (optional)

1 tbsp. vegan butter or popcorn butter (liquid)

Directions:

Add the tbsp. coconut oil to a boiler and heat. Pour Kernels in the heated coconut oil and pop. In a zip lock back add all seasonings pour in melted vegan butter or popcorn butter and mix. Pour seasoning mixture over popcorn and toss until all popcorn is coated.

Coconut Trail Mix

½ cup raisins

½ cup unsweetened coconut flakes

1 cup mixed unsalted nuts

½ cup sunflower seeds

Directions:

Mix ingredients in a bowl.

Frozen Banana Date Honey

4-6 bananas frozen

½ cup chopped nuts (almonds, peanuts, walnuts, or pecans)

2 ½ tbsps. unsweetened coconut

Popsicle sticks

Directions:

Mix date honey and coconut. Peel bananas and insert popsicle sticks. Dip the bananas in the date honey and coconut and roll in the chopped nuts. Press the banana slight to pick up nuts. Align a tray with parchment paper. Place bananas on the paper and freeze for 1-2 hours.

Choco-Banana Pudding

2 bananas, frozen in chunks
2-3 Tbsp. raw cacao
2-4 Tbsp. unsweetened vanilla almond milk
1 Tbsp. chopped toasted almonds or walnuts (optional)

Directions:

Thaw out bananas for 2-3 minutes.
Add bananas, cacao, and almond milk to your blender and pulse until the mixture is blended. Serve in a bowl, top with nuts and sliced bananas

Kale Chips

1 bunch or a bag kale (stemmed removed and tear leaves into pieces)

2 tbsps. extra virgin olive oil (drizzled over kale)

sea salt

1 lemon zest

Direction:

Heat oven 350 degrees

Place kale on a cookie sheet, drizzle with olive oil and sprinkle with sea salt. Rotate the tray once until crisp. Bake for 12-15 minutes. Toss with lemon zest.4

Mix and Match: Get creative with this recipe.

Try flavors over the kale (e.g. cayenne, supreme herb spice, garlic powder, onion powder, paprika)

CHAPTER 11

Stay Hydrated with Infused Water

Infused Water Recipes

Drink infused water to hydrate the body. Blending various flavors can help with flushing body fat, boost energy, and decrease belly fat. Enjoy these recipes to add to your daily weight loss goals and weight maintenance. Refrigerate 12 to 24 hours to get the full enhanced flavor of the infused water.

Blueberry Hill
1-quart water
½ cup blueberries
10 halved sliced strawberries

Lemon Lime
1-quart water

1 sliced orange peeled

½ sliced lemon peeled

½ sliced lime peeled

Lemon Raspberry

1-quart water

½ cup raspberry

½ sliced lemon peeled

4 mint leaves

Apple Pineapple

1-quart water

12 slices pineapple chunks

½ sliced orange peeled

10 slices cantaloupe

Ginger Orange Pineapple

1-quart water

1 tbsp. ground ginger

½ sliced orange peeled

½ cup pineapple chunks

Basil Lemon Strawberry

1-quart water

½ sliced lemon peeled

½ cup strawberries

¼ tsp. fresh or ground basil

Watermelon Pineapple

1-quart water

1 cup watermelon cubed

½ cup pineapple chunks

½ sliced lemon peeled

¼ cup raspberry

Strawberry Orange Raspberry

1-quart water

½ cup sliced strawberries

½ cup raspberry

½ orange slices

Cinnamon Orange Mint

1-quart water

1 tsp. cinnamon

½ sliced orange peeled

6 mint leaves

Pineapple Blueberry

1-quart water

1 cup pineapple chunks

½ blueberries

½ sliced lemon peeled

Raspberry Pineapple

1-quart water

½ cup raspberry

½ pineapple chunks

Blueberry Green Apple

1-quart water

½ cup blueberry

1 sliced green apple

1 sliced lemon

Pineapple Mango Coconut

1-quart coconut water

1 sliced pineapple

1 sliced, peeled mango

Lemon Mint

1 -quart water

1 sliced lemon

5 leaves mint

Cherry Blackberry Lime

1-quart water

5-8 blackberries

5-8 Red cherries

1 sliced lime

Chapter 12

Getting on the Path After the Fast

"Clarity, Vitality, and Serenity Health"

Twenty-one days have passed since you started the Daniel Fast. Now that it is over, you may have dropped a few pounds, committed to eating healthier, gained more energy, your skin has cleared, you feel at peace with your inner beings, or maintained your weight for better health. How did the Daniel Fast help you? Did the fast succeed your expectation? Have you grown spiritually? Is your connection with God more vertically then horizontally?

So, let's recap on the benefits of the Daniel Fast. The Daniel Fast is a self-body fasting cleanser where we are eliminating certain foods for 21-Days. During this time, you usually pray for God to do things you want to see changed in your life and by His Grace it will be done. You may have prayed for better eating habits, healing, spiritual guidance, and intervention. Let me encourage you to continue to pray for these things throughout the year. Keep your ears open to hear His voice and your eyes open to see the move of His hands over your life. Give praises and acknowledge Him always.

I suggested changing your eating habits at the beginning of the book. If you prayed for eating habit changes, that is awesome. This is the time you need to consider a plan that will keep you healthy for the rest of your life just by eating the right foods, exercising, and cutting healthcare cost. I always tell people before making or considering any changes in diet, it's better that you to talk with your physician.

Let me tell you a little about "*A Healthier You Detoxify and Cleanse Program.*" "*A Healthier You*" is a unique detox and cleanse wellness program designed to teach you how to eat healthy and detox the body daily with smoothies, herbal teas, healthy snacks, and meal plans: live well by gaining clarity, vitality, and serenity. This successful detox plan program exceeds beyond expectations because it includes various ways to detox your body even when you are not trying to lose weight.

"A Healthier You" detox and cleanse program will help you to incorporate and manage your eating habits to address many concerns that you may have about healthy living. "A Healthier You Six-Tier Plans" have various options on healthy eating that will help you to detox and cleanse the body. The Six-Tier Plan includes the 10/14 Fit & Smoothie Cleanse, The Ultimate Healing Foods Plan, 14 Day Detox and Cleanse w/Meals Plan, Start Eating 5 Day Meal Plan, 7-Day Allergy Detox and Cleanse, and Detox Life After Maintenance Plan.

"A Healthier You Six Tier Plans" are not used to treat any chronic illnesses or disorders, but will help you build a program that is affordable and durable to gain optimal wellness for your chronic illness, disorder and weight loss. Personal coaching and group coaching is available via my website. You will have access to detox and cleanse plans once you subscribe to the website. When you become a VIP member with "A Healthier You", you will receive several perks such as discounts for conferences, online store purchases, healthy eating management plans, coaching, and free recipes.

****

Services

We offer workshops for school districts for educators, churches, public and private organizations, corporate businesses, and host health and wellness events.

****

A Healthier You w/Dr. V. Benson
21- Day Daniel Fast Recipes

Other Wellness Plans:

3-Day Turbo Intensity Jump Start to weight loss

Healthier Kids Eating Plan

****

Published Book:

"10/14 Fit & Smoothie Cleanse: Unleash the Empowerment to Change Your Lifestyle"

****

See the website for additional information:
http://www.ahealthieryoudetoxify-cleansewithdrvbenson.org

My Additional Prayers and Thoughts Worksheet:

_____

_____

_____

_____

_____

_____

_____

_____

_____

_____

_____

_____

_____

_____

_____

_____

_____

A Healthier You w/Dr. V. Benson
21- Day Daniel Fast Recipes

_____

_____

_____

_____

_____

_____

_____

_____

www.ingramcontent.com/pod-product-compliance
Lightning Source LLC
Chambersburg PA
CBHW070154290526
45789CB00002B/768